Ketogenic Air Fryer Recipes for Everybody

Get in Shape and Lose Weight with Tasty and Affordable Recipes for Beginners

Morgan Parry

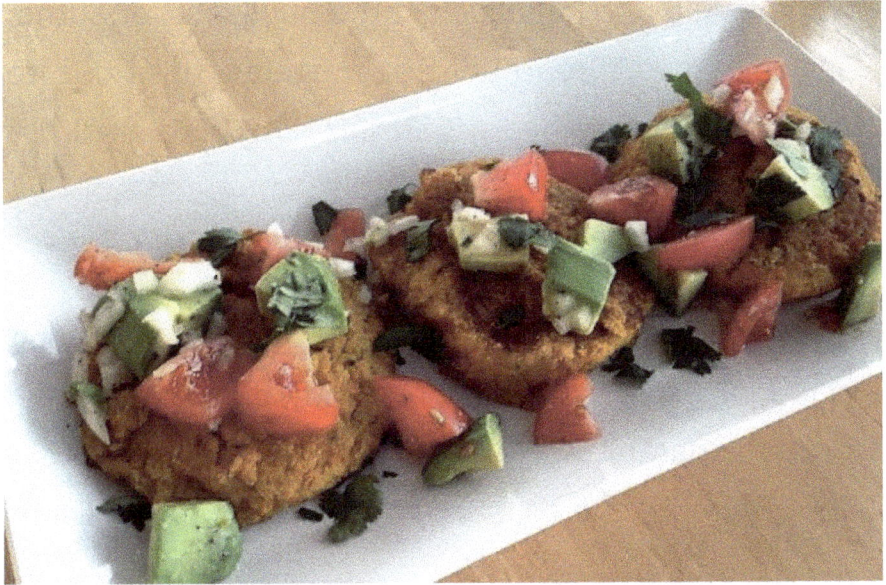

advice. The content within this book has been derived from various sources. Please consult a licensed professional before attempting any techniques outlined in this book.

By reading this document, the reader agrees that under no circumstances is the author responsible for any losses, direct or indirect, which are incurred as a result of the use of information contained within this document, including, but not limited to, — errors, omissions, or inaccuracies.

Table of Contents

Broccoli and Cranberries Mix 10

Coconut Kohlrabi Mash 12

Broccoli and Scallions Sauce... 14

Cheesy Rutabaga 16

Chili Lime Broccoli... 18

Paprika Jicama 19

Parmesan Veggie Mix 22

Squash Noodles 24

Almond Broccoli and Chives... 26

Cayenne Eggplant Puree 28

Butter Broccoli.. 30

Swiss Asparagus.. 31

Lime Kale and Bell Peppers Bowls 33

Okra Salad 36

Balsamic Garlic Kale... 38

Halloumi Skewers.. 39

Coconut Parmesan Kale 42

Creamy Cauliflower 44

Paprika Kale and Olives 46

Roasted Cauliflower.. 47

Coconut Mushrooms Mix 49

Red Vinegar and Chicken Mix.. 51

Oregano and Lemon Chicken Drumsticks... 53

Thyme and Sage Turkey Breasts 56

Onion and Cayenne Chicken Tenders.. 59

Turkey and Butter Sauce 61

Garlic Chicken Sausages 63

Ginger Turkey and Cherry Tomatoes 65

Cayenne and Turmeric Chicken Strips......................... 68

Turkey Stew 70

Turmeric Zucchini Patties... 72

Herbed Asparagus and Sauce 74

Cheesy Green Patties 77

Balsamic Asparagus and Tomatoes.............................. 79

Mozzarella Green Beans 81

Cheddar Asparagus 83

Sesame Fennel.. 84

Mustard Garlic Asparagus.. 86

Mozzarella Asparagus Mix.. 88

Thyme Radish Mix... 89

Paprika Asparagus 91

Nutmeg Okra 93

Lemon Asparagus.. 94

Feta Peppers 95

Spicy Kale 97

Buffalo Broccoli 99

Kale and Sprouts 101

Paprika Leeks.. 103

Coconut Broccoli 105

Zucchini and Squash Mix.. 108

Broccoli and Cranberries Mix

Preparation time: 5 minutes

Cooking time 25 minutes

Serving: 4

Ingredients:

- 1 broccoli head, florets separated 2 shallots, chopped

- A pinch of salt and black pepper

- ½ cup cranberries

- ½ cup almonds, chopped

- 6 bacon slices, cooked and crumbled 3 tablespoons balsamic vinegar

Directions:

1. In a pan that fits the air fryer, combine the broccoli with the rest of the ingredients and toss. Put the pan in the air fryer and cook at 380 degrees F for 25 minutes. Divide between plates and serve.

Nutrition: calories 173, fat 7, fiber 2, carbs 4, protein 8

Coconut Kohlrabi Mash

Preparation time: 10 minutes

Cooking time 20 minute

Serving: 6

Ingredients:

- 12 oz kohlrabi, chopped
- 2 tablespoons coconut cream
- 1 teaspoon salt
- ½ cup Monterey Jack cheese, shredded
- ¼ cup chicken broth
- ½ teaspoon chili flakes

Directions:

1.   In the air fryer pan mix up kohlrabi, coconut cream, salt, Monterey jack cheese, chicken broth, and chili flakes. Then preheat the air fryer to 255F. Cook the meal for 20 minutes.

Nutrition: calories 64, fat 4.2, fiber 2.2, carbs 3.9, protein 3.6

Broccoli and Scallions Sauce

Preparation time: 5 minutes

Cooking time 15 minutes

Serving: 4

Ingredients:

- 1 broccoli head, florets separated Salt and black pepper to the taste

- ½ cup keto tomato sauce

- 1 tablespoon sweet paprika

- ¼ cup scallions, chopped 1 tablespoon olive oil

Directions:

1. In a pan that fits the air fryer, combine the broccoli with the rest of the ingredients, toss, put the pan in the fryer and cook at 380 degrees F for 15 minutes. Divide between plates and serve.

Nutrition: calories 163, fat 5, fiber 2, carbs 4, protein 8

Cheesy Rutabaga

Preparation time: 15 minutes

Cooking time 8 minutes

Serving: 2

Ingredients:

- 6 oz rutabaga, chopped

- 2 oz Jarlsberg cheese, grated

- 1 tablespoon butter

- ½ teaspoon dried parsley

- ½ teaspoon salt

- ½ teaspoon minced garlic

- 3 tablespoons heavy cream

Directions:

1. In the mixing bowl mix up a rutabaga, dried parsley, salt, and minced garlic. Then add heavy cream and mix up the vegetables well. After this, preheat the

air fryer to 375F. Put the rutabaga mixture in the air fryer and cook it for 6 minutes. Then stir it well and top with grated cheese. Cook the meal for 2 minutes more. Transfer the cooked rutabaga in the plates and top with butter.

Nutrition: calories 262, fat 22.4, fiber 2.2, carbs 7.8, protein 8.7

Chili Lime Broccoli

Preparation time: 5 minutes

Cooking time 15 minutes

Serving: 4

Ingredients:

- pound broccoli florets 2 tablespoons olive oil

- tablespoons chili sauce Juice of 1 lime

- A pinch of salt and black pepper

Directions:

1.   In a bowl, mix the broccoli with the other ingredients and toss well. Put the broccoli in your air fryer's basket and cook at 400 degrees F for 15 minutes. Divide between plates and serve.

Nutrition: calories 173, fat 6, fiber 2, carbs 6, protein 8

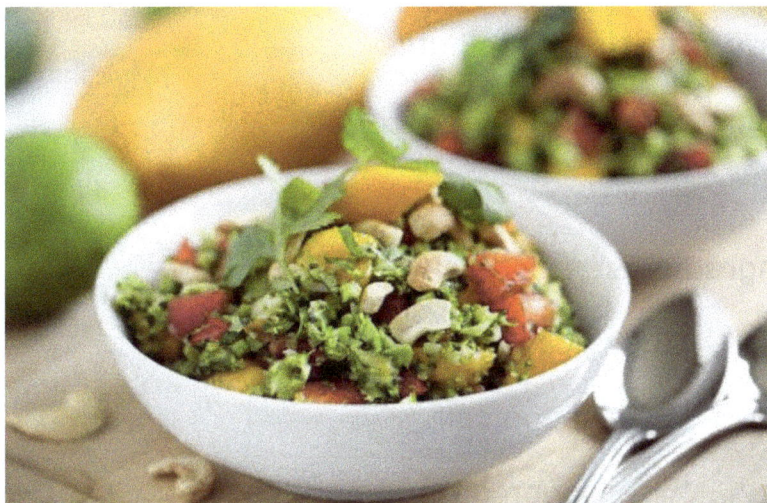

Paprika Jicama

Preparation time: 15 minutes

Cooking time 7 minutes

Serving: 5

Ingredients:

- 15 oz jicama, peeled

- ½ teaspoon salt

- ½ teaspoon ground paprika

- ½ teaspoon chili flakes

- 1 teaspoon sesame oil

Directions:

1.   Preheat the air fryer to 400F. Cut Jicama into the small sticks and sprinkle with salt, ground paprika, and chili flakes. Then put the Jicama stick in the air fryer and sprinkle with sesame oil. Cook the vegetables for 4 minutes. Then shake them well and cook for 3 minutes.

Nutrition: calories 34, fat 0.8, fiber 3.5, carbs 6.4, protein 0.5

Parmesan Veggie Mix

Preparation time: 5 minutes

Cooking time 15 minutes

Serving: 4

Ingredients:

*   1 broccoli head, florets separated

*   ½ pound asparagus, trimmed Juice of 1 lime

*   Salt and black pepper to the taste 2 tablespoons olive oil

*   3 tablespoons parmesan, grated

Directions:

1.   In a bowl, mix the asparagus with the broccoli and all the other ingredients except the parmesan, toss, transfer to your air fryer's basket and cook at 400 degrees F for 15 minutes. Divide between plates, sprinkle the parmesan on top and serve.

Nutrition: calories 172, fat 5, fiber 2, carbs 4, protein 9

Squash Noodles

Preparation time: 20 minutes

Cooking time 5 minutes

Serving: 4

Ingredients:

- 12 oz scallop squash
- 1 teaspoon butter, softened
- 1 oz Parmesan, grated
- 1 teaspoon sesame oil
- ¼ teaspoon cayenne pepper

Directions:

1. Make the noodles from the scallop squash. Use the spiralizer for this step. Then place the vegetable noodles in the air fryer and sprinkle with sesame oil. Cook them for 5 minutes at 385F. Transfer the cooked noodles in the plates and sprinkle with butter and cayenne pepper. Then top the vegetables with Parmesan,

Nutrition: calories 57, fat 3.8, fiber 0, carbs 3.6, protein 3.3

Almond Broccoli and Chives

Preparation time: 5 minutes

Cooking time 12 minutes

Serving: 4

Ingredients:

- 1 pound broccoli florets 3 garlic cloves, minced
- A pinch of salt and black pepper 3 tablespoons coconut oil, melted
- ½ cup almonds, chopped
- 1 tablespoon chives, chopped 2 tablespoons red vinegar

Directions:

1. In a bowl, mix the broccoli with the garlic, salt, pepper, vinegar and the oil and toss. Put the broccoli in your air fryer's basket and cook at 380 degrees F for 12 minutes. Divide between plates and serve with almonds and chives sprinkled on top.

Nutrition: calories 180, fat 4, fiber 2, carbs 4, protein 6

Cayenne Eggplant Puree

Preparation time: 15 minutes **Cooking time** 15 minutes

Serving: 2

Ingredients:

- 1 large eggplant, trimmed, peeled
- 1 teaspoon cayenne pepper
- ¼ cup chicken broth
- 1 garlic clove, peeled
- ½ teaspoon salt
- 1 teaspoon dried parsley
- ½ teaspoon avocado oil

Directions:

1.   Sprinkle the eggplant with salt and avocado oil. Put it in the air fryer and cook for 15 minutes at 390F. Then cool the cooked eggplant gently and chop roughly. Transfer it in the blender. Add chicken broth, cayenne

pepper, garlic, and dried parsley. Grind the mixture until it smooth.

2.   Transfer the cooked meal in the bowl.

Nutrition: calories 69, fat 0.9, fiber 8.4, carbs 14.7, protein 3.1

Butter Broccoli

Preparation time: 5 minutes

Cooking time 15 minutes

Serving: 4

Ingredients:

- pound broccoli florets
- A pinch of salt and black pepper 1 teaspoons sweet paprika
- ½ tablespoon butter, melted

Directions:

1. In a bowl, mix the broccoli with the rest of the ingredients, and toss. Put the broccoli in your air fryer's basket, cook at 350 degrees F for 15 minutes, divide between plates and serve.

Nutrition: calories 130, fat 3, fiber 3, carbs 4, protein 8

Swiss Asparagus

Preparation time: 10 minutes

 Cooking time 6 minutes

Serving: 4

Ingredients:

- 12 oz asparagus, trimmed
- 2 eggs, beaten
- ¼ cup Swiss cheese, shredded
- ½ cup coconut flour
- 1 teaspoon olive oil
- 1 teaspoon salt

Directions:

1.   In the mixing bowl mix up Swiss cheese, coconut flour, and salt. Then dip the asparagus in the beaten eggs and coat in the coconut flour mixture.

2.   Repeat the same steps one more time and transfer the coated asparagus in the air fryer basket. Cook the vegetables for 6 minutes at 395F.

Nutrition: calories 154, fat 7.8, fiber 7.8, carbs 12.8, protein 9.5

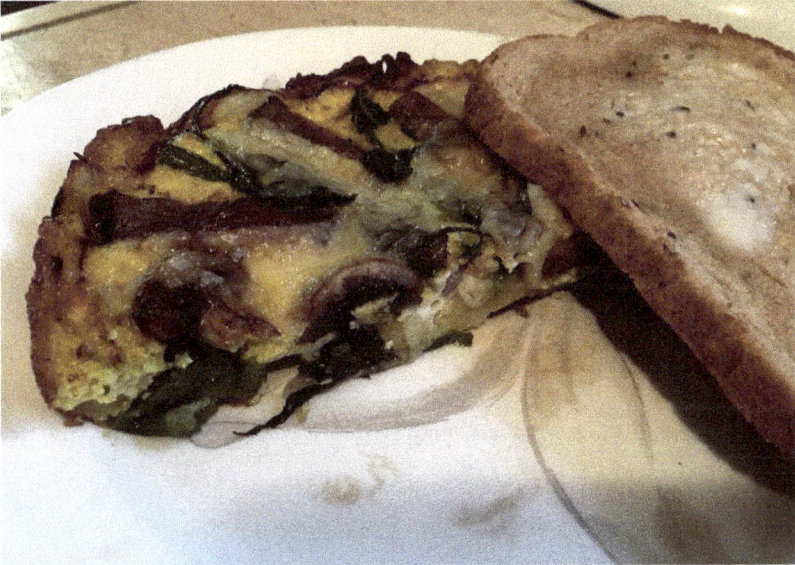

Lime Kale and Bell Peppers Bowls

Preparation time: 5 minutes

Cooking time 10 minutes

Serving: 4

Ingredients:

- cups kale, torn

- A pinch of salt and black pepper

- 1 and ½ cups avocado, peeled, pitted and cubed 1 cup red bell pepper, sliced

- ¼ cup olive oil

- tablespoon mustard

- tablespoons lime juice

- tablespoon white vinegar

Directions:

1. In a pan that fits the air fryer, combine the kale with salt, pepper, avocado and half of the oil, toss, put in

your air fryer and cook at 360 degrees F for 10 minutes. In a bowl, combine the kale mix with the rest of the ingredients, toss and serve.

Nutrition: calories 131, fat 3, fiber 2, carbs 4, protein 5

Okra Salad

Preparation time: 10 minutes

Cooking time 6 minutes

Serving: 2

Ingredients:

- 6 oz okra, sliced

- 3 oz green beans, chopped

- 1 cup arugula, chopped

- 1 teaspoon lemon juice

- 1 teaspoon olive oil

- ½ teaspoon salt

- 2 eggs, beaten

- 1 tablespoon coconut flakes

- Cooking spray

Directions:

1.   In the mixing bowl mix up sliced okra and green beans. Add cooking spray and salt and mix up the mixture well. Then add beaten eggs and shake it. After this, sprinkle the vegetables with coconut flakes and shake okra and green beans to coat them in the coconut flakes. Preheat the air fryer to 400F. Put the vegetable mixture in the air fryer and cook it for 6 minutes. Shake the mixture after 3 minutes of cooking. After this, mix up cooked vegetables with arugula, lemon juice, and sprinkle with olive oil. Shake the salad.

Nutrition: calories 142, fat 7.8, fiber 4.6, carbs 10.5, protein 8.3

Balsamic Garlic Kale

Preparation time: 2 minutes

Cooking time 12 minutes

Serving: 6

Ingredients:

* tablespoons olive oil 3 garlic cloves, minced

* 2 and ½ pounds kale leaves

* Salt and black pepper to the taste 2 tablespoons balsamic vinegar

Directions:

1. In a pan that fits the air fryer, combine all the ingredients and toss. Put the pan in your air fryer and cook at 300 degrees F for 12 minutes. Divide between plates and serve.

Nutrition: calories 122, fat 4, fiber 3, carbs 4, protein 5

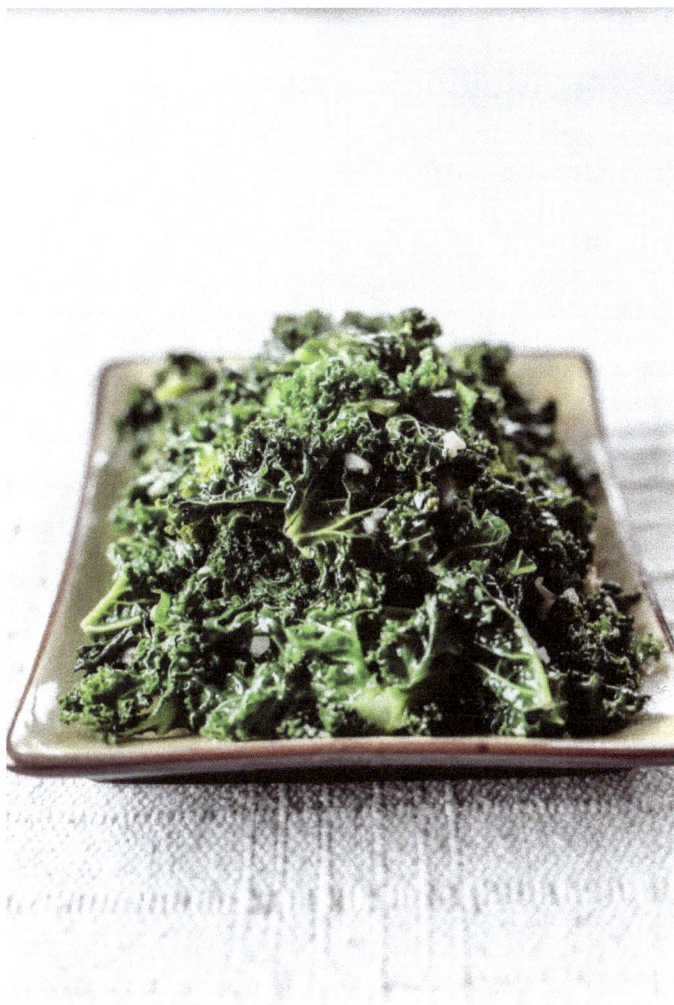

Halloumi Skewers

Preparation time: 15 minutes

Cooking time 14 minutes

Serving: 4

Ingredients:

- 10 oz halloumi cheese
- 1 eggplant
- 1 green bell pepper
- 1 teaspoon dried cilantro
- 1 tablespoon avocado oil
- ½ teaspoon salt
- 1 teaspoon chili flakes

Directions:

1. Chop eggplant, pepper, and eggplant roughly. Then chop halloumi. Put all ingredients from the list above in the big bowl and shake well. Then string the ingredients on the wooden skewers and place in the air

fryer. Cook the kebabs for 14 minutes at 400F. Flip the kebabs on another side after 6 minutes of cooking.

Nutrition: calories 301, fat 21.9, fiber 4.6, carbs 11, protein 16.8

Coconut Parmesan Kale

Preparation time: 5 minutes

Cooking time 15 minutes

Serving: 4

Ingredients:

- 2 pounds kale, torn

- A pinch of salt and black pepper 2 tablespoons olive oil

- 2 garlic cloves, minced

- 1 and ½ cups coconut cream

- ½ teaspoon nutmeg, ground

- ½ cup parmesan, grated

Directions:

1.   In a pan that fits your air fryer, mix the kale with the rest of the ingredients, toss, introduce the pan in the fryer and cook at 400 degrees F for 15 minutes. Divide between plates and serve.

Nutrition: calories 135, fat 3, fiber 2, carbs 4, protein 6

Creamy Cauliflower

Preparation time: 10 minutes

Cooking time 12 minutes

Serving: 4

Ingredients:

- 1-pound cauliflower
- 1 teaspoon taco seasonings
- 1 tablespoon heavy cream
- 1 teaspoon olive oil

Directions:

1.   Chop the cauliflower roughly and sprinkle it with taco seasonings and heavy cream. Then sprinkle the cauliflower with olive oil. Preheat the air fryer to 400F. Cook it for 12 minutes. Shake the vegetables every 3 minutes.

Nutrition: calories 56, fat 2.7, fiber 2.8, carbs 7.1, protein 2.3

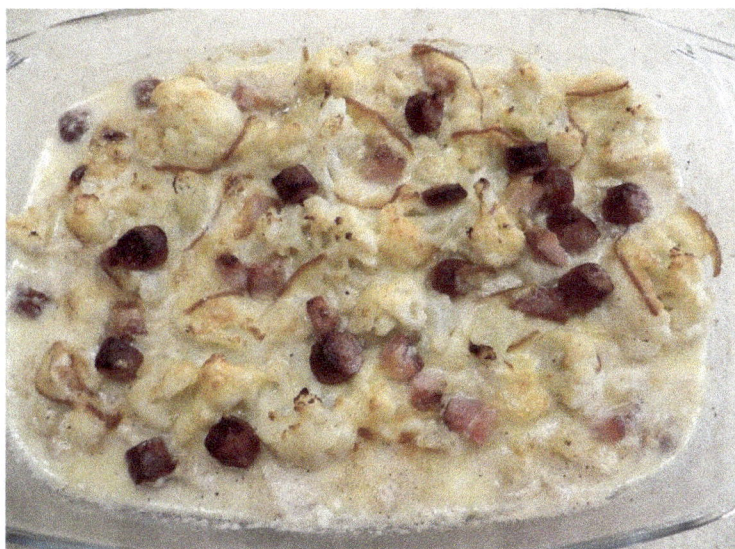

Paprika Kale and Olives

Preparation time: 5 minutes

Cooking time 15 minutes

Serving: 4

Ingredients:

- an ½ pounds kale, torn 2 tablespoons olive oil

- Salt and black pepper to the taste 1 tablespoon hot paprika

- tablespoons black olives, pitted and sliced

Directions:

1. In a pan that fits the air fryer, combine all the ingredients and toss. Put the pan in your air fryer, cook at 370 degrees F for 15 minutes, divide between plates and serve.

Nutrition: calories 154, fat 3, fiber 2, carbs 4, protein 6

Roasted Cauliflower

Preparation time: 15 minutes

Cooking time 25 minutes

Serving: 4

Ingredients:

- 12 oz cauliflower head
- 2 tablespoons butter, melted
- 1 teaspoon ground turmeric
- ½ teaspoon salt
- ¼ teaspoon cayenne pepper
- 1 bacon slice, chopped

Directions:

1. In the mixing bowl mix up butter, ground turmeric, salt, and cayenne pepper Then fill the cauliflower head with chopped bacon. After this, brush the vegetable with melted butter mixture generously. Preheat the air fryer to 365F. Put the cauliflower head in the air fryer basket and cook it for 25 minutes.

Nutrition: calories 100, fat 7.9, fiber 2.3, carbs 5, protein 3.6

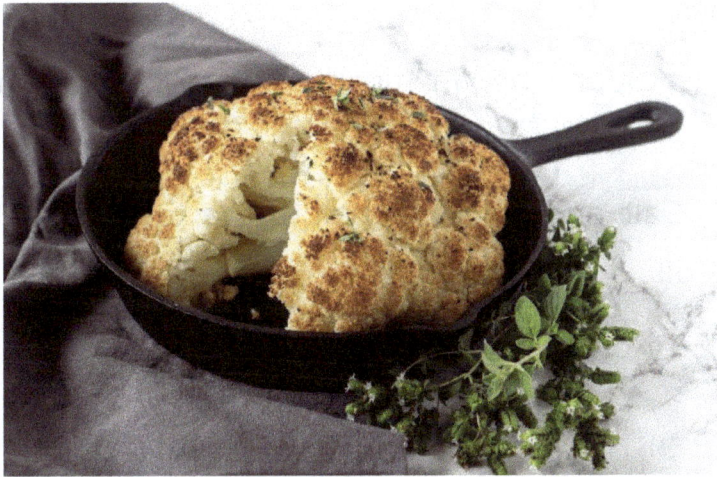

Coconut Mushrooms Mix

Preparation time: 5 minutes

Cooking time 15 minutes

Serving: 4

Ingredients:

- 1 pound brown mushrooms, sliced 1 pound kale, torn

- Salt and black pepper to the taste 2 tablespoons olive oil

- 14 ounces coconut milk

Directions:

1. In a pan that fits your air fryer, mix the kale with the rest of the ingredients and toss. Put the pan in the fryer, cook at 380 degrees F for 15 minutes, divide between plates and serve.

Nutrition: calories 162, fat 4, fiber 1, carbs 3, protein 5

Red Vinegar and Chicken Mix

Preparation time: 5 minutes

Cooking time 30 minutes

Serving: 4

Ingredients:

• pounds chicken wings, halved

• ¼ cup red vinegar

• 4 garlic cloves, minced

• Salt and black pepper to the taste 4 tablespoons olive oil

• tablespoon garlic powder 1 teaspoon turmeric powder

Directions:

1. In a bowl, mix the chicken with all the other ingredients and toss well. Put the chicken wings in your air fryer's basket and cook at 370 degrees F for 30 minutes, flipping the meat halfway. Divide everything between plates and serve with a side salad.

Nutrition: calories 250, fat 12, fiber 4, carbs 6, protein 15

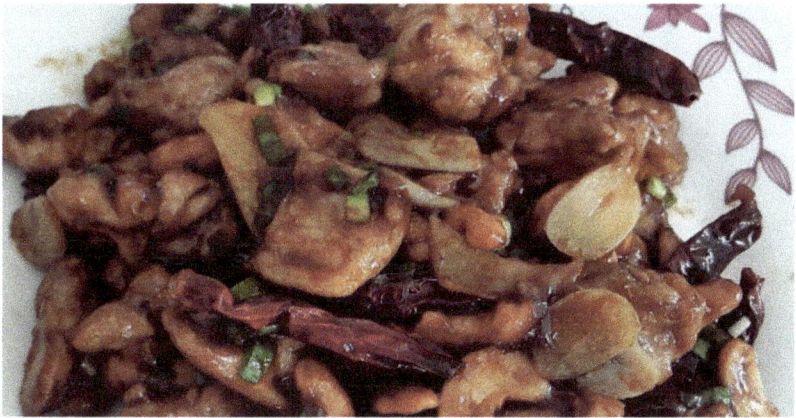

Oregano and Lemon Chicken Drumsticks

Preparation time: 15 minutes

Cooking time 21 minutes

Servings: 4

Ingredients:

- 4 chicken drumsticks, with skin, bone-in

- 1 teaspoon dried cilantro

- ½ teaspoon dried oregano

- ½ teaspoon salt

- 1 teaspoon lemon juice

- 1 teaspoon butter, softened

- 2 garlic cloves, diced

Directions:

1. In the mixing bowl mix up dried cilantro, oregano, and salt. Then fill the chicken drumstick's skin with a cilantro mixture. Add butter and diced garlic. Sprinkle the chicken with lemon juice. Preheat the air fryer to 375F.

Put the chicken drumsticks in the air fryer and cook them for 21 minutes.

Nutrition: calories 89, fat 3.6, fiber 0.1, carbs 0.7, protein 12.8

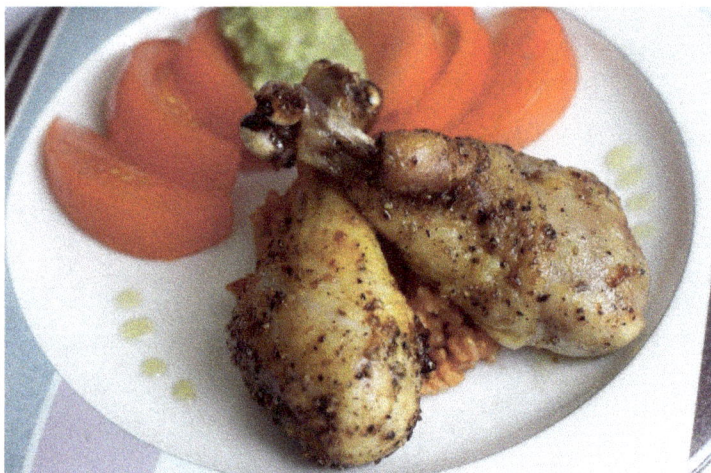

Thyme and Sage Turkey Breasts

Preparation time: 10 minutes

Cooking time 25 minutes

Servings: 4

Ingredients:

• turkey breasts, skinless, boneless and halved 4 tablespoons butter, melted

• 2 tablespoons thyme, chopped 2 tablespoons sage, chopped

• tablespoons rosemary, chopped 2 tablespoons parsley, chopped A pinch of salt and black pepper 2 cups chicken stock

• celery stalks, chopped

Directions:

1.   Heat up a pan that fits your air fryer with the butter over medium-high heat, add the turkey and brown for 2-3 minutes on each side. Add the herbs, stock, celery, salt

and pepper, toss, put the pan in your air fryer, cook at 390 degrees F for 20 minutes. Divide between plates and serve.

Nutrition: calories 284, fat 14, fiber 2, carbs 6, protein 20

Onion and Cayenne Chicken Tenders

Preparation time: 15 minutes

Cooking time 10 minutes

Servings: 2

Ingredients:

- 8 oz chicken fillet

- 1 teaspoon minced onion

- ¼ teaspoon onion powder

- ¼ teaspoon salt

- ½ teaspoon cayenne pepper

- Cooking spray

Directions:

1.   Cut the chicken fillet on 2 tenders and sprinkle with salt, onion powder, and cayenne pepper. Then preheat the air fryer to 365F. Spray the air fryer basket with cooking spray from inside and place the chicken tenders in it. Top the chicken with minced onion and cook for 10 minutes at 365F.

Nutrition: calories 219, fat 8.5, fiber 0.2, carbs 0.7, protein 32.9

Turkey and Butter Sauce

Preparation time: 5 minutes

Cooking time 24 minutes

Servings: 4

Ingredients:

• turkey breast, skinless, boneless and cut into 4 pieces A pinch of salt and black pepper

• Juice of 1 lemon

• tablespoons rosemary, chopped 2 tablespoons butter, melted

Directions:

1. In a bowl, mix the butter with the rosemary, lemon juice, salt and pepper and whisk really well. Brush the turkey pieces with the rosemary butter, put them your air fryer's basket, cook at 380 degrees F for 12 minutes on each side. Divide between plates and serve with a side salad.

Nutrition: calories 236, fat 12, fiber 4, carbs 6, protein 13

Garlic Chicken Sausages

Preparation time: 20 minutes

Cooking time 10 minutes

Servings: 4

Ingredients:

- 1 garlic clove, diced

- 1 spring onion, chopped

- 1 cup ground chicken

- ½ teaspoon salt

- ½ teaspoon ground black pepper

- 4 sausage links

- 1 teaspoon olive oil

Directions:

1.   In the mixing bowl, mix up a diced garlic clove, onion, ground chicken, salt, and ground black pepper. Then fill the sausage links with the ground chicken mixture. Cut every sausage into halves and secure the endings.

2.	Preheat the air fryer to 365. Brush the sausages with olive oil and put it in the air fryer. Cook them for 10 minutes. Then flip the sausages on another side and cook for 5 minutes more. Increase the cooking time to 390F and cook for 8 minutes for faster results.

Nutrition: calories 130, fat 8.3, fiber 0.1, carbs 1, protein 12.2

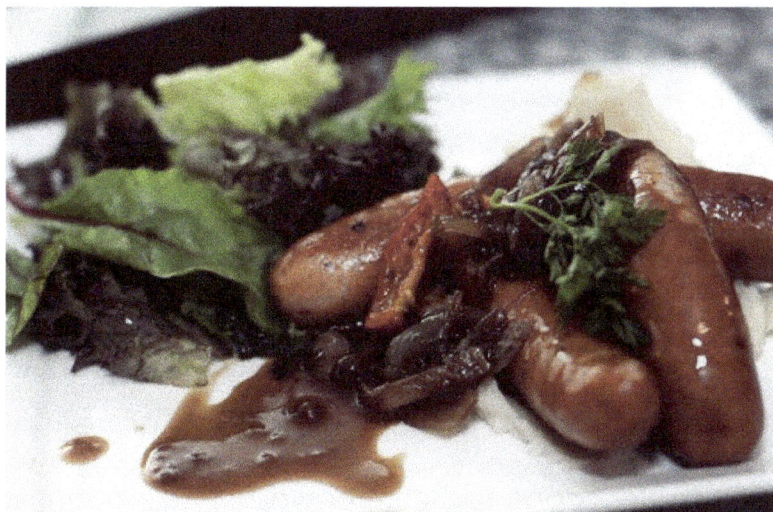

Ginger Turkey and Cherry Tomatoes

Preparation time: 5 minutes

Cooking time 25 minutes

Serving: 4

Ingredients:

- pound turkey breast, skinless, boneless and cubed 1 cup heavy cream

- A pinch of salt and black pepper 4 ounces cherry tomatoes, halved 1 tablespoon ginger, grated

- tablespoons red chili powder 2 teaspoons olive oil

Directions:

1. Heat up a pan that fits the air fryer with the oil over medium heat, add the turkey and brown for 2 minutes on each side. Add the rest of the ingredients, toss, put the pan in the machine and cook at 380 degrees F for 20 minutes. Divide everything between plates and serve.

Nutrition: calories 267, fat 13, fiber 4, carbs 6, protein 16

Cayenne and Turmeric Chicken Strips

Preparation time: 15 minutes

Cooking time 14 minutes

Servings: 6

Ingredients:

- 2-pound chicken breast, skinless, boneless

- 1 teaspoon salt

- 1 teaspoon ground turmeric

- ½ teaspoon cayenne pepper

- 1 egg, beaten

- 2 tablespoons coconut flour

Directions:

1. Cut the chicken breast into the strips and sprinkle with salt, ground turmeric, and cayenne pepper. Then add beaten egg in the chicken strips and stir the mixture. After this, add coconut flour and stir it. Preheat the air fryer to 400F. Put ½ part of all chicken strips in the air

fryer basket in one layer and cook them for 7 minutes. Repeat the same steps with the remaining chicken strips.

Nutrition: calories 195, fat 4.9, fiber 1, carbs 1.7, protein 33.4

Turkey Stew

Preparation time: 5 minutes

Cooking time 25 minutes

Servings: 4

Ingredients:

•   ½ pound brown mushrooms, sliced Salt and black pepper to the taste

•   ¼ cup keto tomato sauce

•   1 turkey breast, skinless, boneless, cubed and browned 1 tablespoon parsley, chopped

Directions:

1.   In a pan that fits your air fryer, mix the turkey with the mushrooms, salt, pepper and tomato sauce, toss, introduce in the fryer and cook at 350 degrees F for 25 minutes. Divide into bowls and serve for lunch with parsley sprinkled on top.

Nutrition: calories 220, fat 12, fiber 2, carbs 5, protein 12

Turmeric Zucchini Patties

Preparation time: 15 minutes

Cooking time 10 minutes

Servings: 4

Ingredients:

- 2 zucchinis, trimmed, grated
- 1 egg yolk
- ½ teaspoon salt
- 1 teaspoon ground turmeric
- ½ teaspoon ground paprika
- 1 teaspoon cream cheese
- 3 tablespoons flax meal
- 1 teaspoon sesame oil

Directions:

1. Squeeze the juice from the zucchinis and put them in the big bowl. Add egg yolk, salt, ground turmeric,

ground paprika, flax meal, and cream cheese. Stir the mixture well with the help of the spoon. Then make medium size patties from the zucchini mixture. Preheat the air fryer to 385F. Brush the air fryer basket with sesame oil and put the patties inside. Cook them for 5 minutes from each side.

Nutrition: calories 67, fat 4.7 fiber 2.8, carbs 5.5, protein 3.1

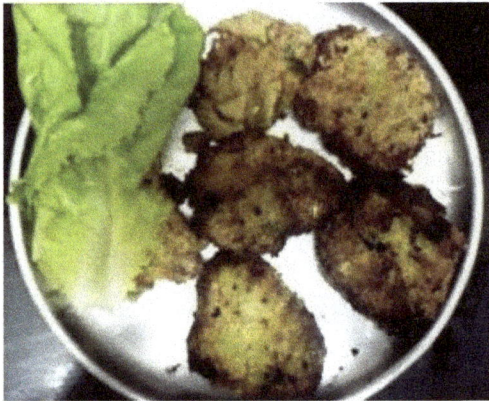

Herbed Asparagus and Sauce

Preparation time: 4 minutes Cooking

time: 10 minutes

Serving: 4

Ingredients:

- 1 pound asparagus, trimmed 2 tablespoons olive oil

- A pinch of salt and black pepper 1 teaspoon garlic powder

- 1 teaspoon oregano, dried 1 cup Greek yogurt

- cup basil, chopped

- ½ cup parsley, chopped

- ¼ cup chives, chopped

- ¼ cup lemon juice

- garlic cloves, minced

Directions:

1.   In a bowl, mix the asparagus with the oil, salt, pepper, oregano and garlic powder, and toss. Put the asparagus in the air fryer's basket and cook at 400 degrees F for 10 minutes. Meanwhile, in a blender, mix the yogurt with basil, chives, parsley, lemon juice and garlic cloves and pulse well. Divide the asparagus between plates, drizzle the sauce all over and serve.

Nutrition: calories 194, fat 6, fiber 2, carbs 4, protein 8

Cheesy Green Patties

Preparation time: 20 minutes

Cooking time 6 minutes

Serving: 2

Ingredients:

- 1 ½ cup fresh spinach, chopped
- 3 oz provolone cheese, shredded
- 1 egg, beaten
- ¼ cup almond flour
- ½ teaspoon salt
- Cooking spray

Directions:

1. Put the chopped spinach in the blender and blend it until you get a smooth mixture. After this, transfer the grinded spinach in the big bowl. Add shredded provolone cheese, beaten egg, almond flour, and salt. Stir the spinach mixture with the help of the spoon until it is homogenous. Then make the patties from the spinach

mixture. Preheat the air fryer to 400F. Spray the air fryer basket with cooking spray from inside and put the spinach patties. Cook them for 3 minutes and then flip on another side.

2.   Cook the patties for 3 minutes more or until they are light brown.

Nutrition: calories 206, fat 15.4, fiber 0.9, carbs 2.7, protein 15

Balsamic Asparagus and Tomatoes

Preparation time: 5 minutes

Cooking time 10 minutes

Servings: 4

Ingredients:

- pound asparagus, trimmed
- cups cherry tomatoes, halved
- ¼ cup parmesan, grated
- ½ cup balsamic vinegar 2 tablespoons olive oil
- A pinch of salt and black pepper

Directions:

1. In a bowl, mix the asparagus with the rest of the ingredients except the parmesan, and toss. Put the asparagus and tomatoes in your air fryer's basket and cook at 400 degrees F for 10 minutes Divide between plates and serve with the parmesan sprinkled on top.

Nutrition: calories 173, fat 4, fiber 2, carbs 4, protein 8

Mozzarella Green Beans

Preparation time: 10 minutes

Cooking time 6 minutes

Serving: 4

Ingredients:

- 1 cup green beans, trimmed
- 2 oz Mozzarella, shredded
- 1 teaspoon butter
- ½ teaspoon chili flakes
- ¼ cup beef broth

Directions:

1. Sprinkle the green beans with chili flakes and put in the air fryer baking pan. Add beef broth and butter. Then top the vegetables with shredded Mozzarella. Preheat the air fryer to 400F. Put the pan with green beans in the air fryer and cook the meal for 6 minutes.

Nutrition: calories 80, fat 3.7, fiber 1.9, carbs 5.8, protein 6.3

Cheddar Asparagus

Preparation time: 5 minutes

Cooking time 10 minutes

Serving: 4

Ingredients:

•   2 pounds asparagus, trimmed 2 tablespoons olive oil

•   1 cup cheddar cheese, shredded 4 garlic cloves, minced

•   4 bacon slices, cooked and crumbled

Directions:

1.   In a bowl, mix the asparagus with the other ingredients except the bacon, toss and put in your air fryer's basket. Cook at 400 degrees F for 10 minutes, divide between plates, sprinkle the bacon on top and serve.

Nutrition: calories 172, fat 6, fiber 2, carbs 5, protein

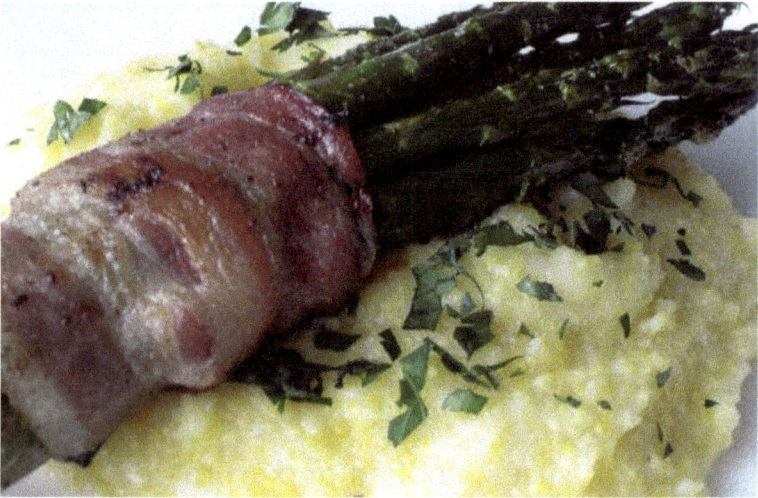

Sesame Fennel

Preparation time: 10 minutes

Cooking time 15 minutes

Serving: 2

Ingredients:

- 8 oz fennel bulb

- 1 teaspoon sesame oil

- ½ teaspoon salt

- 1 teaspoon white pepper

Directions:

1. Trim the fennel bulb and cut it into halves. Then sprinkle the fennel bulb with salt, white pepper, and sesame oil. Preheat the air fryer to 370F. Put the fennel bulb halves in the air fryer and cook them for 15 minutes.

Nutrition: calories 58, fat 2.5, fiber 3.8, carbs 9, protein 1.5

Mustard Garlic Asparagus

Preparation time: 5 minutes

Cooking time 12 minutes

Serving: 4

Ingredients:

• 1 pound asparagus, trimmed 2 tablespoons olive oil

• ¼ cup mustard

• 3 garlic cloves, minced

• ½ cup parmesan, grated

Directions:

1. In a bowl, mix the asparagus with the oil, garlic and mustard and toss really well. Put the asparagus spears in your air fryer's basket and cook at 400 degrees F for 12 minutes. Divide between plates, sprinkle the parmesan on top and serve.

Nutrition: calories 162, fat 4, fiber 4, carbs 6, protein 9

Mozzarella Asparagus Mix

Preparation time: 5 minutes

Cooking time 10 minutes

Serving: 4

Ingredients:

- pound asparagus, trimmed 2 tablespoons olive oil

- A pinch of salt and black pepper 2 cups mozzarella, shredded

- ½ cup balsamic vinegar

- cups cherry tomatoes, halved

Directions:

1. In a pan that fits your air fryer, mix the asparagus with the rest of the ingredients except the mozzarella and toss. Put the pan in the air fryer and cook at 400 degrees F for 10 minutes. Divide between plates and serve.

Nutrition: calories 200, fat 6, fiber 2, carbs 3, protein 6

Thyme Radish Mix

Preparation time: 10 minutes

Cooking time 5 minutes

Serving: 3

Ingredients:

- 2 cups radish, trimmed
- ½ teaspoon onion powder
- ½ teaspoon salt
- ½ teaspoon thyme
- ½ teaspoon ground black pepper
- ½ teaspoon ground paprika
- 1 teaspoon ghee

Directions:

1.   Chop the radish roughly and mix it up with onion powder, salt, thyme, ground black pepper, ad paprika. After this, preheat the air fryer to 375F. Put the roughly chopped radish in the air fryer and cook it for 2 minutes.

Then add ghee, shake well and cook the vegetables for 3 minutes more.

Nutrition: calories 29, fat 1.6, fiber 1.5, carbs 3.5, protein 0.7

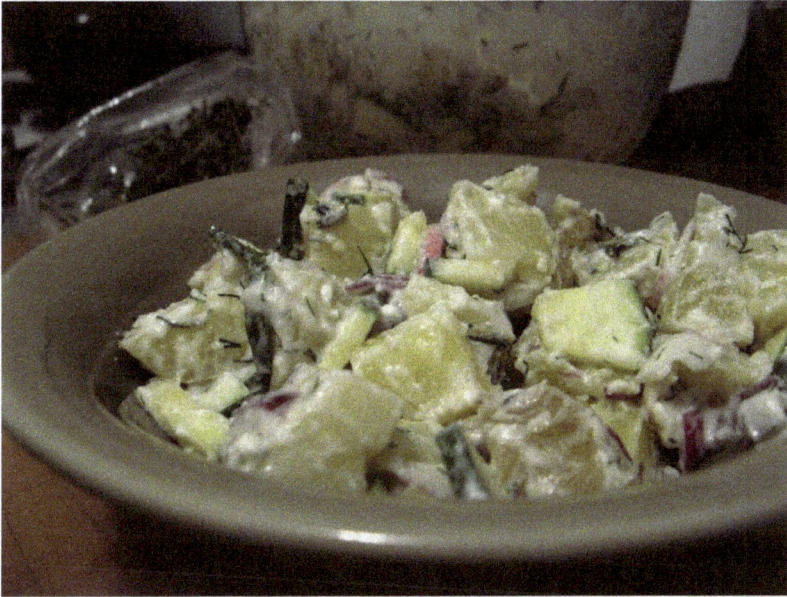

Paprika Asparagus

Preparation time: 5 minutes

Cooking time 10 minutes

Serving: 4

Ingredients:

- 1 pound asparagus, trimmed 3 tablespoons olive oil

- A pinch of salt and black pepper 1 tablespoon sweet paprika

Directions:

1. In a bowl, mix the asparagus with the rest of the ingredients and toss. Put the asparagus in your air fryer's basket and cook at 400 degrees F for 10 minutes. Divide between plates and serve.

Nutrition: calories 200, fat 5, fiber 2, carbs 4, protein 6

Nutmeg Okra

Preparation time: 10 minutes

Cooking time 10 minutes

Serving: 4

Ingredients:

- 1-pound okra, trimmed
- 3 oz pancetta, sliced
- ½ teaspoon ground nutmeg
- ½ teaspoon salt
- 1 teaspoon sunflower oil

Directions:

1. Sprinkle okra with ground nutmeg and salt. Then put the vegetables in the air fryer and sprinkle with sunflower. Chop pancetta roughly. Top the okra with pancetta and cook the meal for 10 minutes at 360F.

Nutrition: calories 172, fat 10.4, fiber 3.7, carbs 8.9, protein 10.1

Lemon Asparagus

Preparation time: 5 minutes

Cooking time 12 minutes

Serving: 4

Ingredients:

- 1 pound asparagus, trimmed
- A pinch of salt and black pepper 2 tablespoons olive oil
- 3 garlic cloves, minced
- 3 tablespoons parmesan, grated Juice of 1 lemon

Directions:

1. In a bowl, mix the asparagus with the rest of the ingredients and toss. Put the asparagus in your air fryer's basket and cook at 390 degrees F for 12 minutes. Divide between plates and serve.

Nutrition: calories 175, fat 5, fiber 2, carbs 4, protein 8

Feta Peppers

Preparation time: 15 minutes

Cooking time 10 minutes

Serving: 4

Ingredients:

- 5 oz Feta, crumbled

- 8 oz banana pepper, trimmed

- 1 teaspoon sesame oil

- 1 garlic clove, minced

- ½ teaspoon fresh dill, chopped

- 1 teaspoon lemon juice

- ½ teaspoon lime zest, grated

Directions:

1. Clean the seeds from the peppers and cut them into halves. Then sprinkle the peppers with sesame oil and put in the air fryer. Cook them for 10 minutes at 385F. Flip the peppers on another side after 5 minutes of cooking. Meanwhile, mix up minced garlic, fresh dill,

lemon juice, and lime zest. Put the cooked banana peppers on the plate and sprinkle with lemon juice mixture. Then top the vegetables with crumbled feta.

Nutrition: calories 107, fat 8.7, fiber 0.2, carbs 2.2, protein 5.2

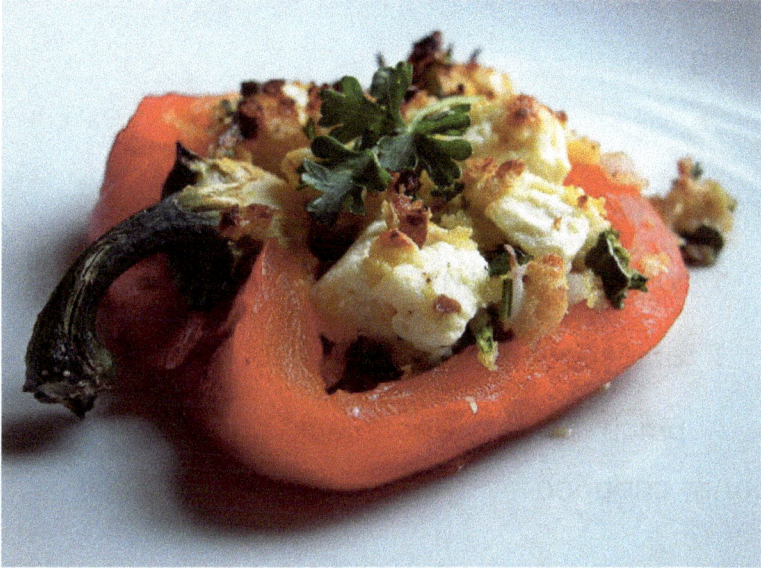

Spicy Kale

Preparation time: 5 minutes

Cooking time 10 minutes

Serving: 4

Ingredients:

•   1 pound kale, torn

•   1 tablespoon olive oil 1 teaspoon hot paprika

•   A pinch of salt and black pepper 2 tablespoons oregano, chopped

Directions:

1.   In a pan that fits the air fryer, combine all the ingredients and toss. Put the pan in the air fryer and cook at 380 degrees F for 10 minutes. Divide between plates and serve.

Nutrition: calories 140, fat 3, fiber 2, carbs 3, protein 5

Buffalo Broccoli

Preparation time: 15 minutes

Cooking time 6 minutes

Serving: 4

Ingredients:

- 2 cups broccoli florets

- ¼ cup of coconut milk

- ½ teaspoon salt

- ½ teaspoon chili flakes

- 1/3 cup coconut flour

- 1 tablespoon Buffalo sauce

- Cooking spray

Directions:

1. Sprinkle the broccoli florets with salt and chili flakes. Then dip them in the coconut milk and coat in the coconut flour. Preheat the air fryer to 400F. Put the broccoli florets in the air fryer, spray with cooking spray, and cook them for 6 minutes. When the broccoli is

cooked, transfer in the bowl and sprinkle with Buffalo sauce.

Nutrition: calories 98, fat 5.4, fiber 5.6, carbs 10.1, protein 3.6

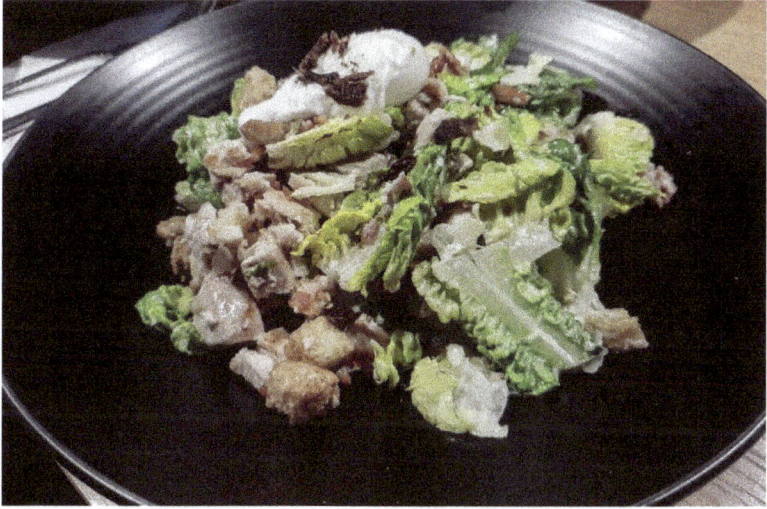

Kale and Sprouts

Preparation time: 5 minutes

Cooking time 15 minutes

Serving: 8

Ingredients:

•   1 pound Brussels sprouts, trimmed 2 cups kale, torn

•   tablespoon olive oil

•   Salt and black pepper to the taste 3 ounces mozzarella, shredded

Directions:

1.   In a pan that fits the air fryer, combine all the ingredients except the mozzarella and toss. Put the pan in the air fryer and cook at 380 degrees F for 15 minutes. Divide between plates, sprinkle the cheese on top and serve.

Nutrition: calories 170, fat 5, fiber 3, carbs 4, protein 7

Paprika Leeks

Preparation time: 15 minutes

Cooking time 8 minutes

Serving: 3

Ingredients:

- 2 big leeks, roughly sliced

- 1 egg, beaten

- ½ teaspoon ground paprika

- ½ teaspoon salt

- ½ teaspoon ground turmeric

- 2 tablespoons almond flour

- Cooking spray

Directions:

1.   Sprinkle the leek slices with ground paprika, salt, and ground turmeric. After this, dip every leek slice in the egg and coat in the almond flour. Preheat the air fryer to 400f and put the leek bites inside. Spray them with

the cooking spray and cook for 8 minutes. Shake after 4 minutes of cooking.

Nutrition: calories 150, fat 10.9, fiber 3.3, carbs 9.2, protein 6.5

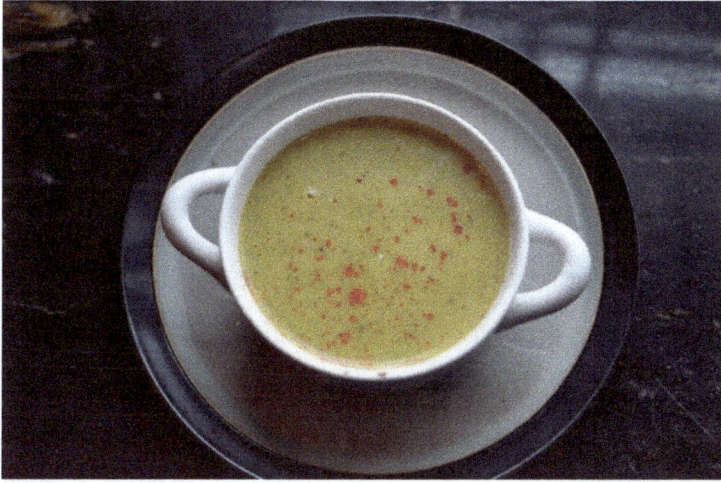

Coconut Broccoli

Preparation time: 5 minutes

Cooking time 30 minutes

Serving: 4

Ingredients:

- 3 tablespoons ghee, melted 15 ounces coconut cream 2 eggs, whisked

- 2 cups cheddar, grated 1 cup parmesan, grated 1 tablespoon mustard

- 1 pound broccoli florets

- A pinch of salt and black pepper 1 tablespoon parsley, chopped

Directions:

1. Grease a baking pan that fits the air fryer with the ghee and arrange the broccoli on the bottom. Add the cream, mustard, salt, pepper and the eggs and toss. Sprinkle the cheese on top, put the pan in the air fryer

and cook at 380 degrees F for 30 minutes. Divide between plates and serve.

Nutrition: calories 244, fat 12, fiber 3, carbs 5, protein 12

Zucchini and Squash Mix

Preparation time: 15 minutes

Cooking time 12 minutes

Serving: 4

Ingredients:

- 10 oz Kabocha squash
- ½ zucchini, chopped
- 3 spring onions, chopped
- 1 teaspoon dried thyme
- 2 teaspoons ghee
- 1 teaspoon salt
- 1 teaspoon ground turmeric

Directions:

1.   Chop the squash into small cubes and sprinkle with salt and ground turmeric. Put the squash in the bowl, add zucchini, spring onions, dried thyme, and ghee. Shake the vegetables gently. Preheat the air fryer to 400F. Put the vegetable mixture in the air fryer and cook for 12

minutes. Shake the vegetables after 6 minutes of cooking to avoid burning.

Nutrition: calories 45, fat 1.8, fiber 1.3, carbs 6.8, protein 1.1

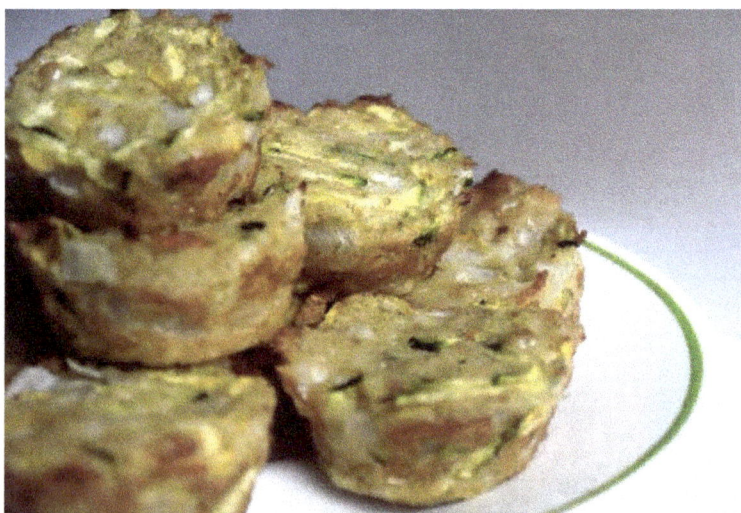

www.ingramcontent.com/pod-product-compliance
Lightning Source LLC
Chambersburg PA
CBHW050751030426
42336CB00012B/1767